Essential Keto Vegetarian Recipes

Easy and Delicious Low-Carb Recipes to Enjoy the Full Benefits of a Plant-Based Ketogenic Diet

Lidia Wong

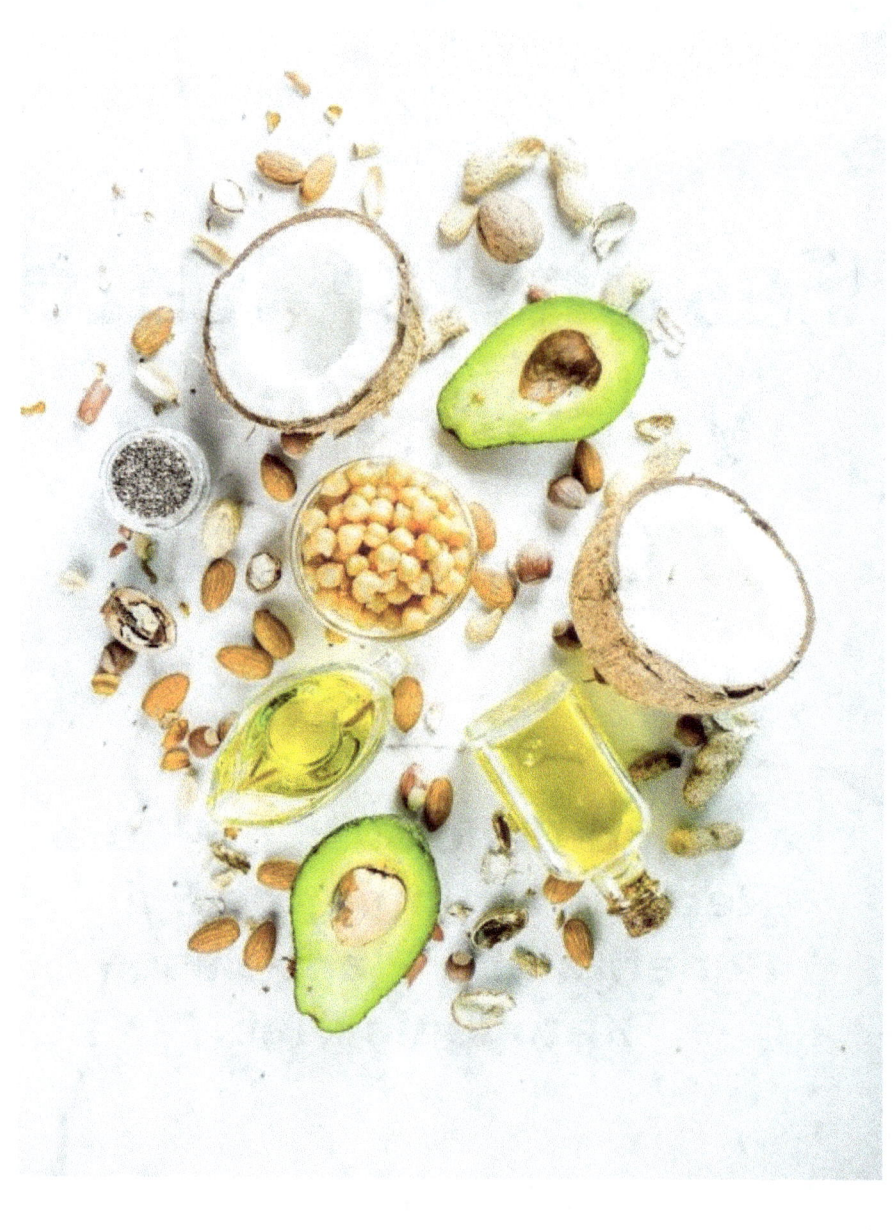

© **Copyright 2021 by Lidia Wong - All rights reserved.**

The content contained within this book may not be reproduced, duplicated or transmitted without direct written permission from the author or the publisher.
Under no circumstances will any blame or legal responsibility be held against the publisher, or author, for any damages, reparation, or monetary loss due to the information contained within this book. Either directly or indirectly.

Legal Notice:
This book is copyright protected. This book is only for personal use. You cannot amend, distribute, sell, use, quote or paraphrase any part, or the content within this book, without the consent of the author or publisher.

Disclaimer Notice:
Please note the information contained within this document is for educational and entertainment purposes only. All effort has been executed to present accurate, up to date, and reliable, complete information. No warranties of any kind are declared or implied. Readers acknowledge that the author is not engaging in the rendering of legal, financial, medical or professional advice. The content within this book has been derived from various sources. Please consult a licensed professional before attempting any techniques outlined in this book.
By reading this document, the reader agrees that under no circumstances is the author responsible for any losses, direct or indirect, which are incurred as a result of the use of information contained within this document, including, but not limited to, — errors, omissions, or inaccuracies.

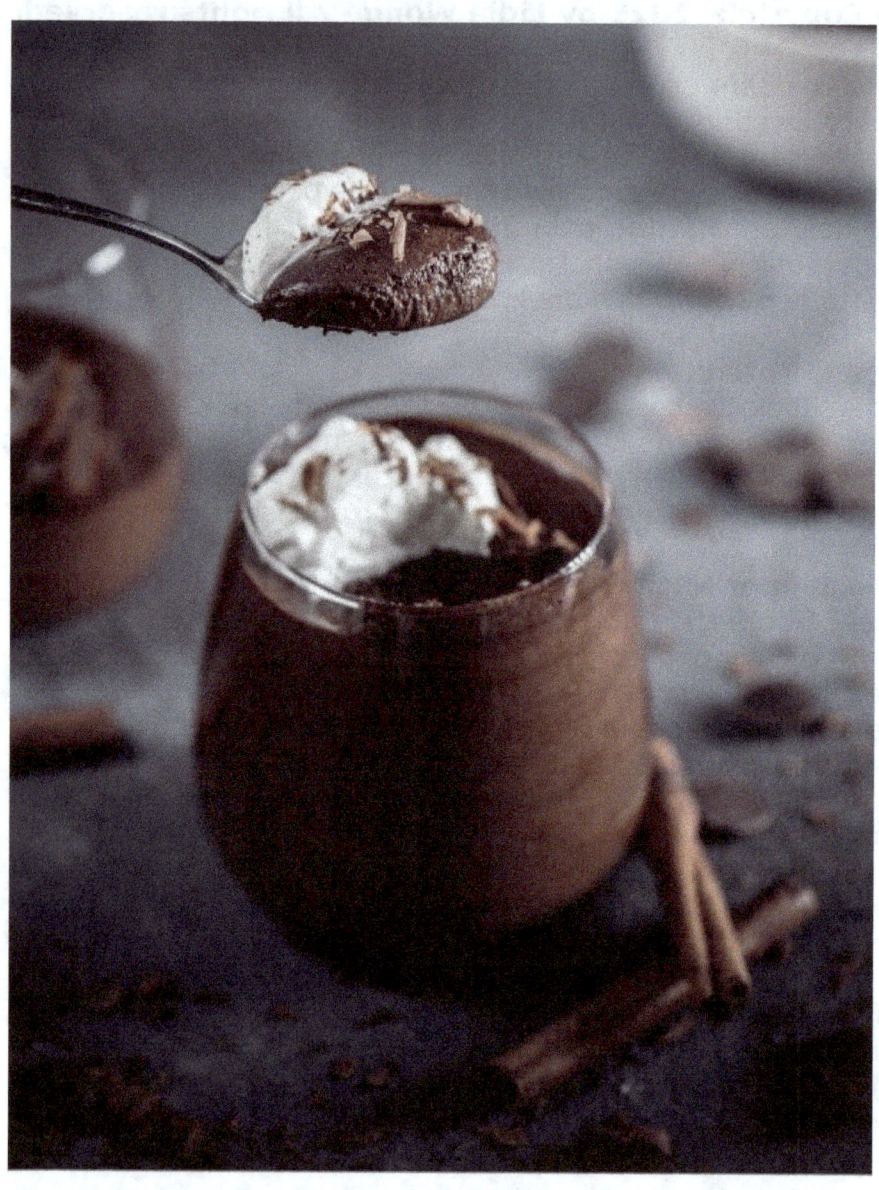

TABLE OF CONTENTS

INTRODUCTION 1

Keto Protein Breakfast Muffins 3

Almond English Muffins 5

Chard Soup 7

Roasted Cauliflower 9

Crustless Veggie Quiche 11

Lime Basil Cucumbers 13

Three Cheese Tofu "Meatza" 14

Baked Mushrooms with Creamy Brussels Sprouts .. 16

Zucchini Boats with Cheese 19

Crunchy Parmesan Crisps 22

Mustard Cabbage Salad 23

Cauliflower Mix 24

Thai Veggie Mix 25

Artichokes with Horseradish Sauce 27

Bok Choy Stir-fry 29

Mustard Greens and Spinach Soup 31

Avocado and Egg Salad 33

Arugula Soup 35

Green Salad 37

Rice And Pea Soup 38

Root Vegetable Bisque 40

Creamy Potato-Cauliflower Soup 42

Zucchini Vegan Bacon Lasagna 44

Pasta & Cheese Mushroom 47

Veggie Medley 51

Gorgonzola 'Blue' Cheese (vegan) 53

Chopped Salad 56

Cucumber-Radish Salad With Tarragon Vinaigrette 58

The Great Green Salad 60

Curried Fruit Salad 61

Potato Salad Redux 63

Brown Rice and Pepper Salad 65

Radish and Walnuts Dip 67

Spinach and Artichoke Dip 69

Chaffles With Raspberry Syrup 71

Banana Chocolate Cupcakes 73

Mint Chocolate Chip Sorbet 75

Pineapple and Melon Stew 77

Pumpkin Spice Oat Bars. 78

Tutti Frutti Cobbler. 80

Bread & Butter Pudding. 82

Pastry with Nuts, Mango and Blueberries 84

Cashew Fudge 86

Raisins and Berries Cream 88

Avocado and Grapes Shake Bowls 89

Avocado Cookies 90

Rice Pudding 92

Strawberry Sorbet 93

Coconut Cream 94

Brown Fat Bombs 95

Nut Fudge 97

Quick Choco Brownie 99

NOTE **101**

INTRODUCTION

The keto diet is the shortened term for ketogenic diet and it is essentially a high-fat and low-carb diet that helps you lose weight, thereby bringing various health benefits. This diet drastically restricts your carb intake while increasing your fat intake; this pushes your body to go into a state know as "*ketosis*". We will tackle ketosis in a bit.

The human body uses glucose from carbs to fuel metabolic pathways—meaning various bodily functions like digestion, breathing, etc.. Essentially, anything that needs energy. Even when you are resting, the body needs fuel or energy for you to continue living. If you think about it, when have you ever stopped breathing, or your heart stopped beating, or your liver stopped from cleansing the body, or your kidneys from filtering blood?

Never, unless you're dead, which is the only time in which the body doesn't need energy. In normal circumstances, glucose is the primary pathway when it comes to sourcing the body's energy.

But the body also has another pathway; it can utilize fats to fuel the various bodily processes. And this is what we call "*ketosis*". And the body can only enter ketosis when there is no glucose available, thus the reason for sticking to a low-carb diet is essential in the keto diet. Since no glucose is available, the body is pushed to use fats—it can either come from the food you consume or from your body's fat reserves—the adipose tissue or from the flabby parts of your body. This is how the keto diet helps you lose weight, by burning up all those stored fats that you have and using it to fuel bodily processes.

That said, if for whatever reason you are a vegetarian, following a ketogenic diet can be extremely difficult. A vegetarian diet is largely free of animal products, which means that food tends to be usually high in carbohydrates. Still, with careful planning, it is possible. This Cookbook will provide you with various easy and delicious dishes to help you stick to your ketogenic diet plan while being a vegetarian.

Enjoy!

Keto Protein Breakfast Muffins

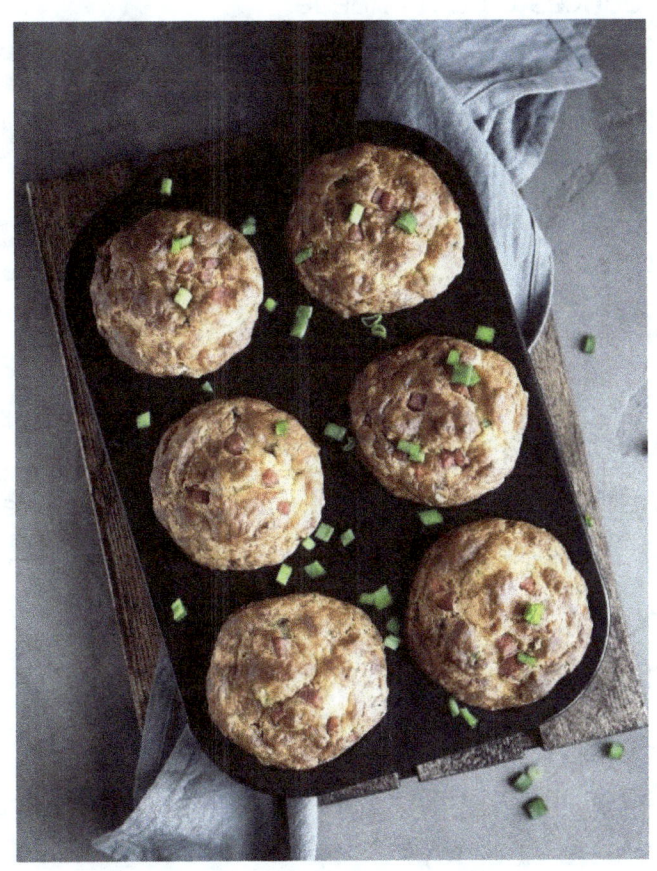

Preparation Time: 12 minutes

Cooking Time: 25 minutes

Servings: 12

Ingredients:

- 8 organic eggs
- 8-ounces cream cheese
- 2 scoops protein powder
- 4 tablespoons butter, melted

Directions:

1. Mix cream cheese and melted butter in a mixing bowl.
2. Add eggs and protein powder and mix well.
3. With the use of a hand mixer mix until well combined and spray your muffin pan with cooking spray.
4. Fill each muffin cup ¾ full of mixture.
5. Bake for 25 minutes in preheated oven at 350°Fahrenheit.
6. Serve and enjoy!

Nutritional Values: (Per Serving):

Calories: 148 Fat: 12.3 g Carbohydrates: 2 g Sugar: 0.4 g Protein: 7.8 g Cholesterol: 116 mg

Almond English Muffins

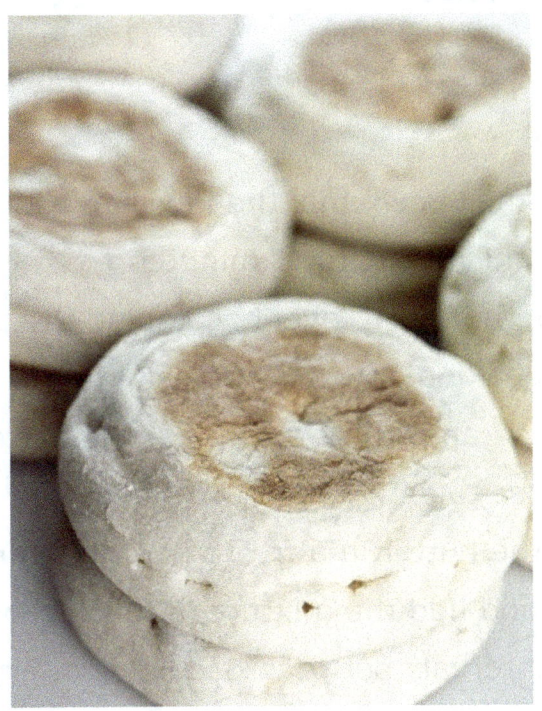

Preparation Time: 10 minutes

Cooking Time: 10 minutes

Serving: 4

Ingredients:

- 2 tbsp almond flour
- 2 tbsp flax seed powder + 6 tbsp water

- ½ tsp baking powder
- 1 pinch salt
- 3 tbsp butter

Directions:

1. In a small bowl, mix the flaxseed with water and allow thickening for 5 minutes.
2. In another bowl, evenly combine the almond flour, baking powder, and salt. Then, pour in the flax egg and whisk again. Let the batter sit for 5 minutes to set.
3. Melt the butter in a frying pan over medium heat and add the mixture in four dollops with 1-inch intervals between each dollop. Fry until golden brown on one side, flip with a spatula and fry further until golden brown.
4. Plate the muffins and serve warm.

Nutrition:

Calories: 263, Total Fat: 26.4g, Saturated Fat:9.5 g, Total Carbs: 4 g, Dietary Fiber: 4g, Sugar:3 g, Protein:4 g, Sodium: 826mg

Chard Soup

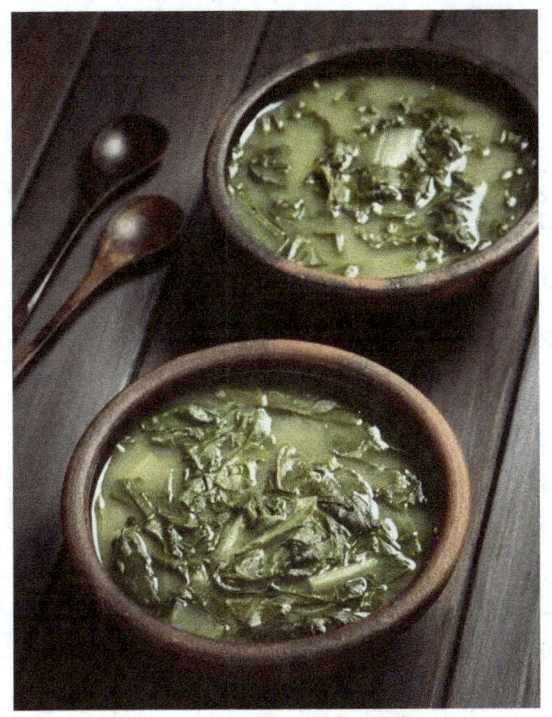

Preparation time: 10 minutes

Cooking time: 25 minutes

Servings: 4

Ingredients:
- 1 pound Swiss chard, chopped
- ½ cup shallots, chopped

- 1 teaspoon cumin, ground
- 1 tablespoon avocado oil
- 1 teaspoon rosemary, dried
- 1 teaspoon basil, dried
- 2 garlic cloves, minced
- Salt and black pepper to the taste
- 6 cups vegetable stock
- 1 tablespoon tomato passata
- 1 tablespoon cilantro, chopped

Directions:

1. Heat up a pan with the oil over medium heat, add the shallots and the garlic and sauté for 5 minutes.
2. Add the Swiss chard and the other ingredients, toss, bring to a simmer and cook over medium heat for 20 minutes more.
3. Divide the soup into bowls and serve.

Nutrition:

Calories 232, fat 23, fiber 3, carbs 4, protein 3

Roasted Cauliflower

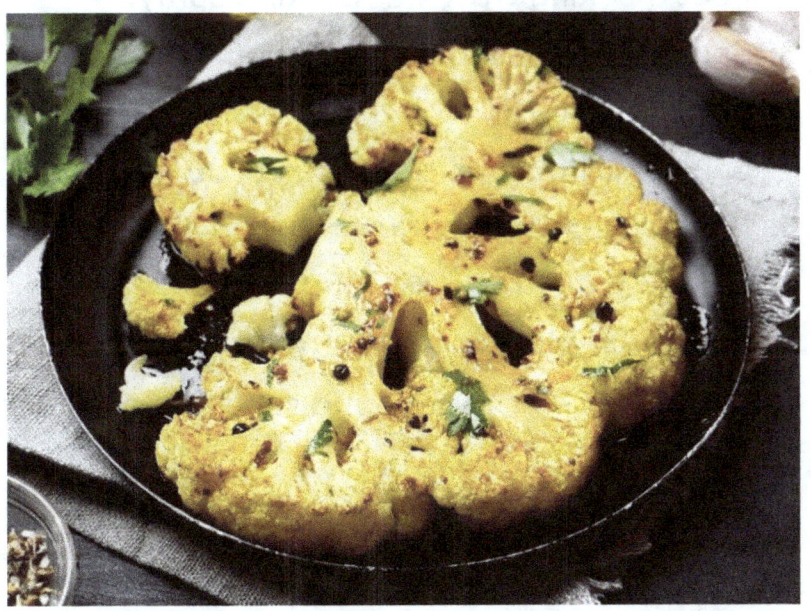

Preparation Time: 10 minutes

Cooking Time: 30 minutes

Servings: 4

Ingredients:

- 1 cauliflower head, cut into florets
- 2 tablespoons fresh sage, chopped
- 1 tablespoon extra-virgin olive oil
- 1 garlic clove, minced

Directions:

1. Preheat your oven to 400°Fahrenheit.
2. Coat a baking tray with cooking spray.
3. Spread the cauliflower florets on the prepared baking tray.
4. Bake cauliflower in the oven for 30 minutes.
5. Meanwhile, sauté garlic in a pan with one tablespoon of olive oil.
6. Remove from heat and set aside.
7. Add cauliflower, garlic, and sage to a bowl and toss to mix.
8. Serve and enjoy!

Nutritional Values (Per Serving):

Calories: 87 Cholesterol: 0 mg Sugar: 5.1 g
Carbohydrates: 12 g Fat: 3.8 g Protein: 4.3 g

Crustless Veggie Quiche

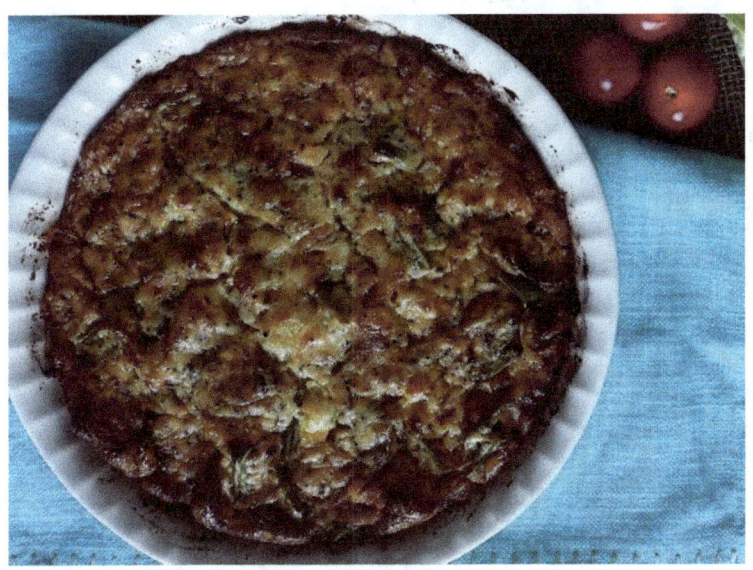

Preparation Time: 10 minutes

Cooking Time: 30 minutes

Servings: 6

Ingredients:
- 1 cup zucchini, chopped
- 1 cup Parmesan cheese, grated, fresh
- 1 cup tomatoes, chopped
- 1 onion, chopped
- 1 cup milk

- 8 eggs, organic
- ½ teaspoon pepper
- 1 teaspoon sea salt

Directions:

1. Preheat your oven to 400°Fahrenheit.
2. In a pan placed over medium heat, melt butter, add onion and sauté until lightly brown.
3. Add zucchini and tomatoes to pan and sauté for 5 minutes.
4. Beat eggs with milk, cheese, pepper and salt in a bowl.
5. Pour egg mixture over veggies and bake in preheated oven for 30 minutes.
6. Allow the dish to cool for 10 minutes, cut into slices, serve and enjoy!

Nutritional Values (Per Serving):

Calories: 257 Sugar: 4.2 g Fat: 16.7 g Carbohydrates: 8.1 g Cholesterol: 257 mg Protein: 21.4 g

Lime Basil Cucumbers

Preparation Time: 15 minutes

Servings: 4

Ingredients:

- 2 medium cucumber, remove seeds and diced
- 1 tsp basil leaves, chopped
- 2 tsp turmeric powder
- 1 tsp fresh lime juice
- 2 tbsp coconut oil
- 1/4 tsp sea salt

Directions:

1. Heat coconut oil in a pan over medium heat.
2. Once the oil is hot then, add turmeric powder and basil leaves and stir for 1 minute.
3. Now add cucumber, lime juice, and salt. Stir well.
4. Serve and enjoy.

Nutritional Value (Amount per Serving):

Calories 85 Fat 7 g Carbohydrates 6 g Sugar 2 g Protein 1 g Cholesterol 0 mg

Three Cheese Tofu "Meatza"

Preparation Time: 10 minutes

Cooking Time: 20 minutes

Serving: 4

Ingredients:

- 1 ½ lb tofu, pressed and crumbled
- Salt and black pepper to taste
- 1 large egg
- 1 tsp thyme
- 3 garlic cloves, minced
- ¼ cup shredded Pecorino Romano cheese
- 1 tsp rosemary
- 1 tsp basil
- ½ tbsp oregano
- ¾ cup low-carb tomato sauce
- 1 cup shredded Monterey Jack cheese
- 1 cup shredded mozzarella cheese

Directions:

1. Preheat the oven to 350 °F and lightly grease a medium pizza pan with cooking spray. Set aside.
2. In a large bowl, mix the tofu, salt, black pepper, egg, thyme, garlic, rosemary, basil, and oregano.
3. Transfer the mixture onto the pizza pan and use your hands to flatten the mix onto the pan with 2-inch thickness. Place in the oven and bake for 15 minutes or until the tofu cooks with a light brown crust.
4. Remove the pizza pan and spread the tomato sauce on top.
5. Scatter the three cheeses one after the other on top and bake further in the oven until the cheeses melt, 5 minutes.
6. Remove the "meatza" from the oven, slice, and serve

Nutrition:

Calories:301, Total Fat: 25.1g, Saturated Fat: 6.7g, Total Carbs: 5g, Dietary Fiber:1 g, Sugar: 2g, Protein: 15g, Sodium: 669mg

Baked Mushrooms with Creamy Brussels Sprouts

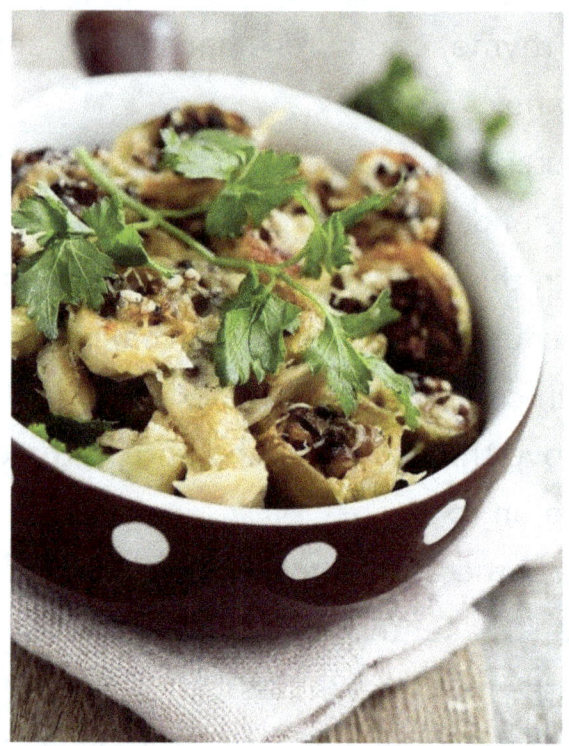

Preparation Time: 8 minutes

Cooking Time: 2 hours 35 minutes

Serving: 4

Ingredients:

For the mushrooms:

- 1 lb whole white button mushrooms
- Salt and black pepper to taste
- 1 bay leaf
- 2 tsp dried thyme
- 5 black peppercorns
- ½ cups vegetable broth
- 2 garlic cloves, minced
- 1 ½ oz fresh ginger, grated
- 1 tbsp coconut oil
- 1 tbsp smoked paprika

For the creamy Brussel sprouts:

- 1 ½ cups cashew cream
- ½ lb Brussel sprouts, halved
- Salt and ground black pepper to taste

Directions:

For the mushroom roast:

1. Preheat the oven to 200 °F.
2. Pour all the mushroom Ingredients into a baking dish, stir well, and cover with foil. Bake in the oven until softened, 1 to 2 hours.

3. Remove the dish, take off the foil, and use a slotted spoon to fetch the mushrooms onto serving plates. Set aside.

For the creamy Brussel sprouts:

4. Pour the broth in the baking dish into a medium pot and add the Brussel sprouts.
5. Add about ½ cup of water if needed and cook for 7 to 10 minutes or until softened.
6. Stir in the cashew cream, adjust the taste with salt and black pepper, and simmer for 15 minutes.
7. Serve the creamy Brussel sprouts with the mushrooms.

Nutrition:

Calories: 492, Total Fat: 37.9g, Saturated Fat: 9.1g, Total Carbs: 13g, Dietary Fiber:2 g, Sugar:2 g, Protein: 29g, Sodium: 779mg

Zucchini Boats with Cheese

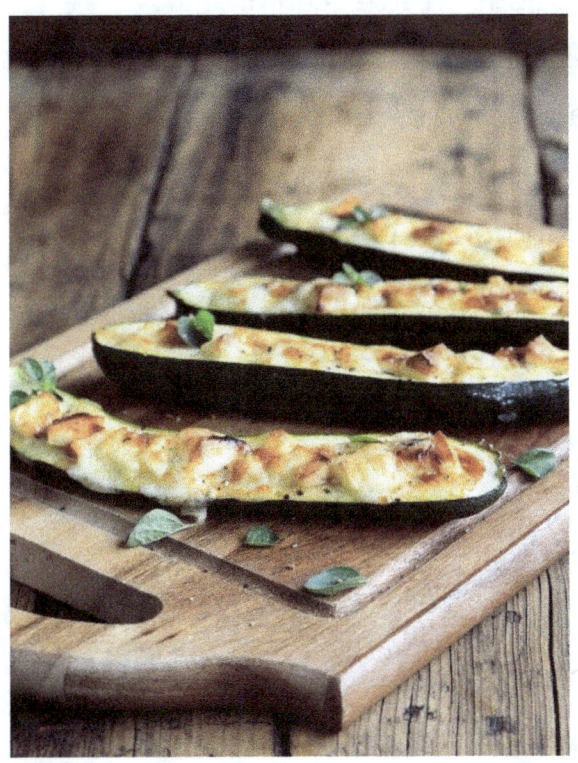

Preparation Time: 3minutes

Cooking Time: 4minutes

Serving: 2

Ingredients:

- 1 cup cheese
- 1 medium-sized zucchini
- 4 tbsp butter
- 2 garlic cloves, minced
- 1½ oz. baby kale
- Salt and black pepper to taste
- 2 tbsp unsweetened tomato sauce
- Olive oil for drizzling

Directions:

1. Preheat the oven to 375 °F.
2. Use a knife to slice the zucchini in halves and scoop out the pulp with a spoon into a plate. Keep the flesh.
3. Grease a baking sheet with cooking spray and place the zucchini boats on top.
4. Put the butter in a skillet and melt over medium heat. Add and sauté the garlic until fragrant and slightly browned, about 4 minutes.
5. Add the kale and the zucchini pulp. Cook until the kale wilts; season with salt and black pepper.

6. Spoon the tomato sauce into the boats and spread to coat the bottom evenly. Then, spoon the kale mixture into the zucchinis and sprinkle with the cheese.
7. Bake in the oven for 20 to 25 minutes or until the cheese has a beautiful golden color.
8. Plate the zucchinis when ready, drizzle with olive oil, and season with salt and black pepper.
9. Serve immediately.

Nutrition:

Calories:721, Total Fat:76.8g, Saturated Fat:21.2g, Total Carbs: 2g, Dietary Fiber:0g, Sugar:0g, Protein:9g, Sodium:309mg

Crunchy Parmesan Crisps

Preparation Time: 5 minutes

Cooking Time: 3 minutes

Servings: 12

Ingredients:

- 12 tablespoons Parmesan cheese, shredded

Directions:

1. Preheat your oven to 400° Fahrenheit.
2. Spray a baking tray with cooking spray.
3. Place each tablespoon of cheese on a baking tray.
4. Bake in preheated oven for 3 minutes or until lightly brown.
5. Allow cooling time, serve and enjoy!

Nutrition:

Calories: 64 Carbohydrates: 0.7 g Sugar: 0 g Fat: 4.3 g Cholesterol: 14 mg Protein: 6.4 g

Mustard Cabbage Salad

Preparation time: 10 minutes

Cooking time: 0 minutes

Servings: 4

Ingredients:

- 1 green cabbage head, shredded
- 1 red cabbage head, shredded
- 2 tablespoons avocado oil
- 1 tablespoon balsamic vinegar
- 2 tablespoons mustard
- 1 teaspoon hot paprika
- Salt and black pepper to the taste
- 1 tablespoon dill, chopped

Directions:

1. In a bowl, mix the cabbage with the oil, mustard and the other ingredients, toss, divide between plates and serve as a side salad.

Nutrition:

Calories 150, fat 3, fiber 2, carbs 2, protein 7

Cauliflower Mix

Preparation time: 10 minutes

Cooking time: 25 minutes

Servings: 4

Ingredients:

- 1 pound cauliflower florets
- 2 tablespoons avocado oil
- 1 teaspoon nutmeg, ground
- 1 tablespoon pumpkin seeds
- 1 teaspoon hot paprika
- 1 tablespoon chives, chopped
- A pinch of sea salt and black pepper

Directions:

1. Spread the cauliflower florets on a baking sheet lined with parchment paper, add the oil, the nutmeg and the other ingredients, toss and bake at 380 degrees F for 25 minutes.
2. Divide the cauliflower mix between plates and serve as a side dish.

Nutrition:

Calories 160, fat 3, fiber 2, carbs 9, protein 4

Thai Veggie Mix

Preparation time: 10 minutes

Cooking time: 3 hours

Servings: 8

Ingredients:

- 8 ounces yellow summer squash, peeled and roughly chopped
- 2 leeks, sliced
- 12 ounces zucchini, halved and sliced
- 2 cups button mushrooms, quartered
- 1 red sweet potatoes, chopped
- 2 tablespoons veggie stock
- 2 garlic cloves, minced
- 2 tablespoon Thai red curry paste
- 1 tablespoon ginger, grated
- ¼ cup basil, chopped
- 1/3 cup coconut milk

Directions:

1. In your slow cooker, mix zucchini with summer squash, mushrooms, red pepper, leeks, garlic, stock, curry paste, ginger, coconut milk and basil, toss, cover and cook on Low for 3 hours.
2. Stir your Thai mix one more time, divide between plates and serve as a side dish.
3. Enjoy!

Nutrition:

Calories 69, fat 2, fiber 2, carbs 8, protein 2

Artichokes with Horseradish Sauce

Preparation time: 10 minutes

Cooking time: 45 minutes

Servings: 2

Ingredients:

- 1 tablespoon horseradish, prepared
- 2 tablespoons mayonnaise
- A pinch of sea salt
- 1 teaspoon lemon juice
- 3 cups artichoke hearts
- Black pepper to taste
- 1 tablespoon lemon juice

Directions:

1. In a bowl, mix horseradish with mayo, a pinch of sea salt, black pepper and 1 teaspoon lemon juice, whisk well and leave aside for now.
2. Arrange artichoke hearts on a lined baking sheet, drizzle 2 tablespoons olive oil over them, 1 tablespoon lemon juice and sprinkle a pinch of salt and some black pepper.

3. Toss to coat well, place in the oven at 425 degrees F and roast for 45 minutes.
4. Divide artichoke hearts between plates and serve with the horseradish sauce on top.
5. Enjoy!

Nutritional value/serving:

Calories 107, fat 5, fiber 3,3, carbs 14,9, protein 1,7

Bok Choy Stir-fry

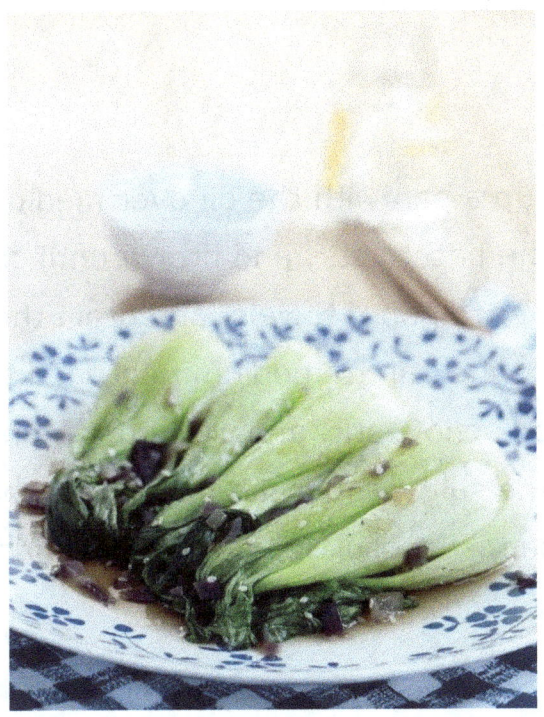

Preparation time: 10 minutes

Cooking time: 7 minutes

Servings: 2

Ingredients:

- 2 cup bok choy, chopped
- 2 garlic cloves, peeled and minced

- 2 bacon slices, chopped
- Salt and ground black pepper, to taste
- A drizzle of avocado oil

Directions:

1. Heat up a pan with the oil over medium heat, add the bacon, stir, and brown until crispy, transfer to paper towels, and drain the grease.
2. Return the pan to medium heat, add the garlic and bok choy, stir, and cook for 4 minutes.
3. Add the salt, pepper, and return the bacon to the pan, stir, cook for 1 minute, divide on plates, and serve.

Nutrition:

Calories - 50, Fat - 1, Fiber - 1, Carbs - 2, Protein - 2

Mustard Greens and Spinach Soup

Preparation time: 10 minutes

Cooking time: 15 minutes

Servings: 6

Ingredients:

- ½ teaspoon fenugreek seeds
- 1 teaspoon cumin seeds
- 1 tablespoon avocado oil
- 5 cups mustard greens, chopped
- 1 cup onion, chopped
- 1 teaspoon coriander seeds
- 1 tablespoon garlic, minced
- 1 tablespoon fresh ginger, grated
- ½ teaspoon turmeric
- 3 cups coconut milk
- 1 tablespoon jalapeño, chopped
- 5 cups spinach, torn
- Salt and ground black pepper, to taste
- 2 teaspoons butter
- ½ teaspoon paprika

Directions:

1. Heat up a pot with the oil over medium-high heat, add the coriander, fenugreek, and cumin seeds, stir, and brown them for 2 minutes.
2. Add the onions, stir, and cook for 3 minutes. Add half of the garlic, jalapeños, ginger, and turmeric, stir, and cook for 3 minutes.
3. Add the mustard greens, and spinach, stir, and sauté everything for 10 minutes.
4. Add the milk, salt, and pepper, and blend the soup using an immersion blender.
5. Heat up a pan with the butter over medium heat, add the garlic, and paprika, stir well, and take off the heat.
6. Heat up the soup over medium heat, ladle into soup bowls, drizzle with butter and sprinkle with paprika all over, and serve.

Nutrition:

Calories - 143, Fat - 6, Fiber - 3, Carbs - 7, Protein - 7

Avocado and Egg Salad

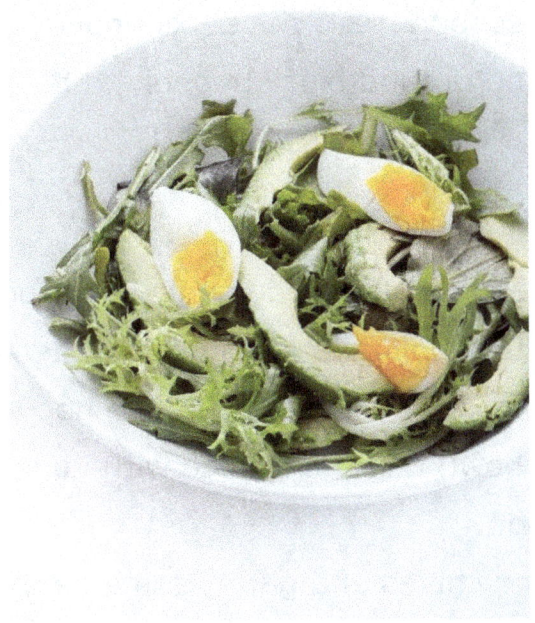

Preparation time: 10 minutes

Cooking time: 7 minutes

Servings: 4

Ingredients:
- 4 eggs
- 4 cups mixed lettuce leaves, torn

- 1 avocado, pitted, and sliced
- ¼ cup mayonnaise
- 2 teaspoons mustard
- 2 garlic cloves, peeled and minced
- 1 tablespoon fresh chives, chopped
- Salt and ground black pepper, to taste

Directions:

1. Put water in a pot, add some salt, add the eggs, bring to a boil over medium-high heat, boil for 7 minutes, drain, cool, peel, and chop them. In a salad bowl, mix the lettuce with eggs, and avocado.
2. Add the chives and garlic, some salt, and pepper, and toss to coat.
3. In a bowl, mix the mustard with mayonnaise, salt, and pepper, and stir well.
4. Add this to the salad, toss well, and serve.

Nutrition:

Calories - 234, Fat - 12, Fiber - 4, Carbs - 7, Protein - 12

Arugula Soup

Preparation time: 10 minutes

Cooking time: 13 minutes

Servings: 6

Ingredients:

- 1 onion, peeled and chopped
- 1 tablespoon olive oil
- 2 garlic cloves, peeled and minced
- 10 ounces baby arugula
- ½ cup coconut milk
- 2 tablespoons fresh mint, chopped, and
- 2 tablespoons fresh tarragon, chopped
- 2 tablespoons fresh parsley, chopped
- 2 tablespoons fresh chives, chopped
- 4 tablespoons coconut milk yogurt
- 6 cups chicken stock
- Salt and ground black pepper, to taste

Directions:

1. Heat up a pot with the oil over medium-high heat, add the onion and garlic, stir, and cook for 5 minutes.
2. Add the stock, and milk, stir, and bring to a simmer.
3. Add the arugula, tarragon, parsley, and mint, stir, and cook for 6 minutes.
4. Add the coconut yogurt, salt, pepper, and chives, stir, cook for 2 minutes, divide into soup bowls, and serve.

Nutrition:

Calories - 200, Fat - 4, Fiber - 2, Carbs - 6, Protein - 10

Green Salad

Preparation time: 10 minutes

Cooking time: 0 minutes

Servings: 4

Ingredients:

- 1 bunch Swiss chard, chopped
- 24 green grapes, halved
- 1 avocado, pitted, peeled, and cubed
- Salt and ground black pepper, to taste
- 2 tablespoons avocado oil
- 1 tablespoon mustard
- 7 sage leaves, chopped
- 1 garlic clove, peeled and minced

Directions:

1. In a salad bowl, mix the Swiss chard with the grapes and avocado cubes.
2. In a bowl, mix the mustard with the oil, sage, garlic, salt, and pepper, and whisk.
3. Add this to the salad, toss to coat well, and serve.

Nutrition:

Calories - 120, Fat - 2, Fiber - 1, Carbs - 4, Protein - 5

Rice And Pea Soup

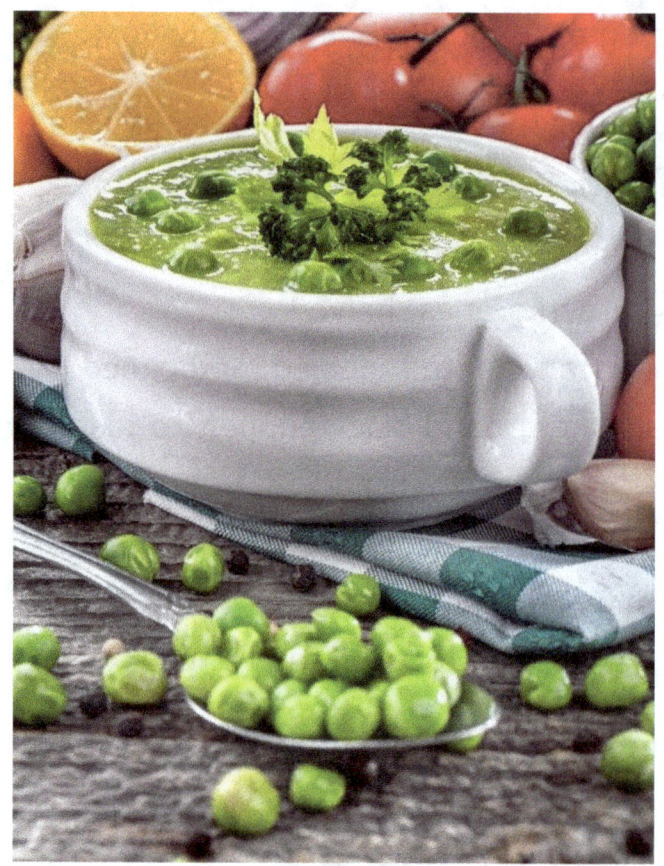

Preparation time: 5 minutes

cooking time: 45 minutes

servings: 4

Ingredients

- 2 tablespoons olive oil
- 1 medium onion, minced
- 2 garlic cloves minced
- 1 cup Arborio rice
- Salt and freshly ground black pepper
- 6 cups vegetable broth, homemade (see Light Vegetable Broth or store-bought, or water
- 1 (16-ouncebag frozen petite green peas
- 1/4 cup chopped fresh flat-leaf parsley

Directions

1. In a large soup pot, heat the oil over medium heat. Add the onion and garlic, cover, and cook until softened for about 5 minutes.
2. Uncover and add the rice, broth, and salt and pepper to taste. Bring to a boil, then reduce heat to low. Cover and simmer until the rice begins to soften, about 30 minutes.
3. Stir in the peas and cook, uncovered, for 15 to 20 minutes longer. Stir in the parsley and serve.

Root Vegetable Bisque

Preparation time: 5 minutes

cooking time: 35 minutes

servings: 4 to 6

Ingredients

- 1 tablespoon olive oil
- 3 large shallots, chopped
- 2 large carrots, shredded
- 2 garlic cloves, minced
- 2 medium parsnips, shredded
- 1 medium potato, peeled and chopped
- 1/2 teaspoon dried thyme
- 1/4 teaspoon dried marjoram
- 1 cup plain unsweetened soy milk
- 4 cups vegetable broth, homemade (see Light Vegetable Broth or store-bought, or water
- Salt and freshly ground black pepper
- 1 tablespoon minced fresh parsley, garnish

Directions

1. In a large soup pot, heat the oil over medium heat.
2. Add the shallots, carrots, parsnips, potato, and garlic.
3. Cover and cook until softened, about 5 minutes.
4. Add the thyme, marjoram, and broth and bring to a boil.
5. Reduce heat to low and simmer, uncovered, until the vegetables are tender, about 30 minutes.
6. Puree the soup in the pot with an immersion blender or in a blender or food processor in batches if necessary, then return to the pot.
7. Stir in the soy milk and taste, adjusting seasonings if necessary.
8. Heat the soup over low heat until hot.
9. Ladle into bowls, sprinkle with parsley, and serve.

Creamy Potato-Cauliflower Soup

Preparation Time: 10 Minutes

Cooking Time: 25 Minutes

Servings: 6

Ingredients

- 1 teaspoon olive oil
- 1 onion, chopped
- 3 cups chopped cauliflower
- 1 or 2 scallions, white and light green parts only, sliced
- 2 potatoes, scrubbed or peeled and chopped
- 6 cups water or Economical Vegetable Broth
- 2 tablespoons dried herbs
- Freshly ground black pepper
- Salt

Directions

1. Heat the olive oil in a large soup pot over medium-high heat.
2. Add the onion and cauliflower, and sauté for about 5 minutes, until the vegetables are

slightly softened.

3. Add the potatoes, water, and dried herbs, and season to taste with salt and pepper.
4. Bring the soup to a boil, reduce the heat to low, and cover the pot.
5. Simmer for 15 to 20 minutes, until the potatoes are soft.
6. Using a hand blender, purée the soup until smooth. (Alternatively, let it cool slightly, then transfer to a countertop blender.)
7. Stir in the scallions and serve.
8. Leftovers will keep in an airtight container for up to 1 week in the refrigerator or up to 1 month in the freezer.

Nutrition Per Serving (2 cups)

Calories: 80; Protein: 2g; Total fat: 1g; Saturated fat: 0g; Carbohydrates: 17g; Fiber: 3g

Zucchini Vegan Bacon Lasagna

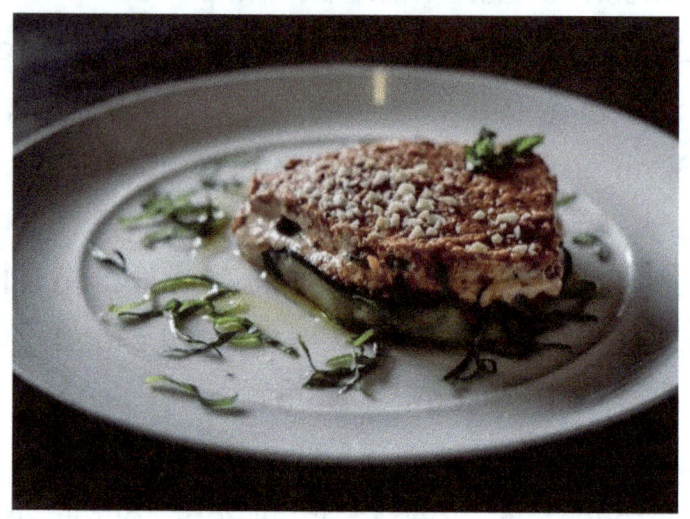

Preparation Time: 15 minutes

Cooking Time: 40 minutes

Serving: 4

Ingredients:

- 4 large yellow zucchinis
- 1 tbsp lard
- ½ lb vegan bacon
- 1 tsp garlic powder
- 1 large egg
- 1 tsp onion powder

- Salt and black pepper to taste
- 2 tbsp coconut flour
- 1 ½ cup grated mozzarella cheese
- 1/3 cup cheddar cheese
- 2 cups crumbled ricotta cheese
- 2 cups unsweetened marinara sauce
- 1 tbsp Italian herb seasoning
- ¼ tsp red chili flakes
- ¼ cup fresh basil leaves

Directions:

1. Preheat the oven to 375 °F and grease a 9 x 9-inch baking dish with cooking spray. Set aside.
2. Slice the zucchini into ¼ -inch strips, arrange on a flat surface and sprinkle generously with salt. Set aside to release liquid for 5 to 10 minutes. Pat dry with a paper towel and set aside.
3. Melt the lard in a large skillet over medium heat and add the vegan bacon. Cook until browned, 10 minutes. Set aside to cool.
4. In a medium bowl, evenly combine the garlic powder, onion powder, coconut flour, salt, black pepper, mozzarella cheese, half of the cheddar cheese, ricotta cheese, and egg. Set aside.

5. Add the Italian herb seasoning and red chili flakes to the marinara sauce and mix. Set aside.
6. Make a single layer of the zucchini in the baking dish; spread a quarter of the egg mixture on top, and a quarter of the marinara sauce. Repeat the layering process and sprinkle the top with the remaining cheddar cheese.
7. Bake in the oven for 30 minutes or until golden brown on top.
8. Remove the dish from the oven, allow cooling for 5 to 10 minutes, garnish with the basil leaves, slice and serve.

Nutrition:

Calories:417, Total Fat: 36.4g, Saturated Fat: 15.9g, Total Carbs: 4g, Dietary Fiber:0g, Sugar: 1g, Protein20: g, Sodium: 525mg

Pasta & Cheese Mushroom

Preparation Time: 1 hour 45 minutes + overtime chilling

Serving size: 4

Ingredients:

For the keto macaroni:

- 1 egg yolk
- 1 cup shredded mozzarella cheese

For the pulled mushroom mac and cheese:

- 2 tbsp olive oil
- 1 lb mushroom
- 1 tsp dried thyme
- 1 cup vegetable broth
- 2 tbsp butter
- 2 medium shallots, minced
- 2 garlic cloves, minced
- Salt and black pepper to taste
- 1 cup water
- 1 cup grated cheddar cheese
- 4 oz dairy- free cream cheese, room temperature

- 1 cup coconut cream
- ½ tsp white pepper
- ½ tsp nutmeg powder
- 2 tbsp chopped parsley

Directions:

For the keto macaroni:

1. Pour the cheese into a medium safe-microwave bowl and melt in the microwave for 35 minutes or until melted.
2. Take out the bowl and allow cooling for 1 minute only to warm the cheese but not cool completely. Mix in the egg yolk until well-combined.
3. Lay a parchment paper on a flat surface, pour the cheese mixture on top and cover with another parchment paper. Using a rolling pin, flatten the dough into 1/8-inch thickness.
4. Take off the parchment paper and cut the dough into small cubes of the size of macaroni. Place in a bowl and refrigerate overnight.
5. When ready to cook, bring 2 cups of water to a boil in a medium saucepan and add the keto macaroni. Cook for 40 seconds to 1 minute and

then drain through a colander. Run cold water over the pasta and set it aside to cool.

For the mushroom mac and cheese:

6. Heat the olive oil in a large pot, season the mushroom with salt, black pepper, thyme, and sear in the oil on both sides until brown. Pour on the vegetable broth, cover, and cook over low heat for 15 minutes or until softened. When ready, remove the mushroom onto a plate and set it aside.
7. Preheat the oven to 380 °F.
8. Melt the butter in a large skillet and sauté the shallots until softened. Stir in the garlic and cook until fragrant, 30 seconds.
9. Pour in the water to deglaze the pot and then stir in half of the cheddar cheese and dairy-free cream cheese until melted, 4 minutes. Mix in the coconut cream and season with salt, black pepper, white pepper, and nutmeg powder.
10. Add the pasta, mushroom, and half of the parsley to the mixture; combine well.
11. Pour the mixture into a baking dish and cover the top with the remaining cheddar cheese.

Bake in the oven until the cheese melts and the food bubbly, 15 to 20 minutes.
12. Remove from the oven, allow cooling for 2 minutes and garnish with the parsley.
13. Serve warm.

Nutrition:

Calories:647, Total Fat:56.5g, Saturated Fat:32g, Total Carbs:6g, Dietary Fiber:1g, Sugar:2g, Protein:30g, Sodium:609mg

Veggie Medley

Preparation time: 10 minutes

Cooking time: 4 hours

Servings: 6

Ingredients:

- 1 tablespoon ginger, grated
- 3 garlic cloves, minced
- 1 yellow onion, chopped
- 4 cups cauliflower florets
- 2 carrots, chopped
- 1 date, pitted and chopped
- 1 and ½ teaspoon coriander, ground
- 1 and ¼ teaspoon cumin, ground
- ½ teaspoon dry mustard
- A pinch of salt and black pepper
- ½ teaspoon turmeric powder
- 1 tablespoon white wine vinegar
- ¼ teaspoon cardamom, ground
- 1 and ½ cups kidney beans, cooked
- 2 zucchinis, chopped
- 6 ounces tomato paste
- 1 green bell pepper, chopped

- 1 cup green peas

Directions:

1. In your slow cooker, mix ginger with garlic, date, coriander, dry mustard, cumin, salt, pepper, turmeric, vinegar, cardamom, carrots, onion, cauliflower, kidney beans, zucchinis, tomato paste, bell pepper and peas, stir, cover and cook on High for 4 hours.
2. Divide into bowls and serve hot.
3. Enjoy!

Nutrition:

Calories 165, fat 2, fiber 10, carbs 32, protein 9

Gorgonzola 'Blue' Cheese (vegan)

Preparation time: 24 hours

Cooking time: 20 minutes

Servings: 16

Ingredients:

- ½ cup macadamia nuts (unsalted)
- ½ cup pine nuts
- 1 cup raw cashews (unsalted)
- 1 capsule acidophilus (probiotic cheese culture)
- ½ tbsp. MCT oil
- ¼ cup unsweetened almond milk
- 1 tsp. Himalayan salt
- 1 tsp. ground black pepper
- 1 tsp. spirulina powder

Directions:

1. Cover the cashews with water in a small bowl and let sit for 4 to 6 hours. Rinse and drain the cashews after soaking. Make sure no water is left.

2. Preheat the oven to 350°F / 175°C, and line a baking sheet with parchment paper.
3. Spread the macadamia and pine nuts out on the baking sheet so they can roast evenly.
4. Put the baking sheet into the oven and roast the nuts for 8 minutes, until they are slightly browned.
5. Take the nuts out of the oven and allow them to cool down.
6. Grease a 3-inch cheese mold with the MCT oil and set it aside.
7. Add all ingredients—except the spirulina—to the blender or food processor. Blend on medium speed into a smooth mixture. Use a spatula to scrape down the sides of the blender to make sure all the ingredients get incorporated.
8. Transfer the cheese mixture into the greased cheese mold and sprinkle it with the spirulina powder. Use a small teaspoon to create blue marble veins on the cheese, and then cover the mold with parchment paper.
9. Place the cheese into a dehydrator and dehydrate the cheese at 90°F / 32°C for 24 hours.

10. Transfer the dehydrated cheese in the covered mold to the fridge. Allow the cheese to refrigerate for 12 hours.
11. Remove the cheese from the mold to serve in this condition, or, age the cheese in a wine cooler for up to 3 weeks. In case of aging the cheese, rub the outsides of the cheese with fresh sea salt. Refresh the salt every 2 days to prevent any mold. The cheese will develop a blue cheese-like taste, and by aging it, the cheese becomes even more delicious.
12. If the cheese is not aged, store it in airtight container and consume within 6 days.
13. Store the aged cheese in an airtight container and consume within 6 days, or for a maximum of 60 days in the freezer and thaw at room temperature.

Nutrition:

Calories: 101kcal, Net Carbs: 2g, Fat: 9.3g, Protein: 2.3g, Fiber: 1g, Sugar: 0.9g

Chopped Salad

Preparation time: 15 minutes

cooking time: 0 minutes

servings: 4

Ingredients

- ¾ cup olive oil
- 1/4 cup white wine vinegar
- 2 teaspoons Dijon mustard
- 1 garlic clove
- 1 tablespoon minced green onions
- 1/2 teaspoon salt (optional
- 1/4 teaspoon ground black pepper
- 1/2 small head romaine lettuce, chopped
- 1/2 small head iceberg lettuce, chopped
- 11/2 cups cooked or 1 (15.5-ouncecan chickpeas, drained and rinsed
- 2 ripe tomatoes, cut into 1/2-inch dice
- 1 medium English cucumber, peeled, halved lengthwise, and chopped
- 2 celery ribs, chopped celery
- 1 medium carrot, chopped
- 1/2 cup halved pitted kalamata olives

- 1 ripe Hass avocado, pitted, peeled, and cut into 1/2-inch dice
- 3 small red radishes, chopped
- 2 tablespoons chopped fresh parsley

Directions

1. In a blender or food processor, combine the oil, vinegar, mustard, garlic, green onions, salt, and pepper.
2. Blend well and set aside.
3. In a large bowl, combine the romaine and iceberg lettuces.
4. Add the chickpeas, tomatoes, cucumber, celery, carrot, olives, radishes, parsley, and avocado.
5. Add enough dressing to lightly coat.
6. Toss gently to combine and serve.

Cucumber-Radish Salad With Tarragon Vinaigrette

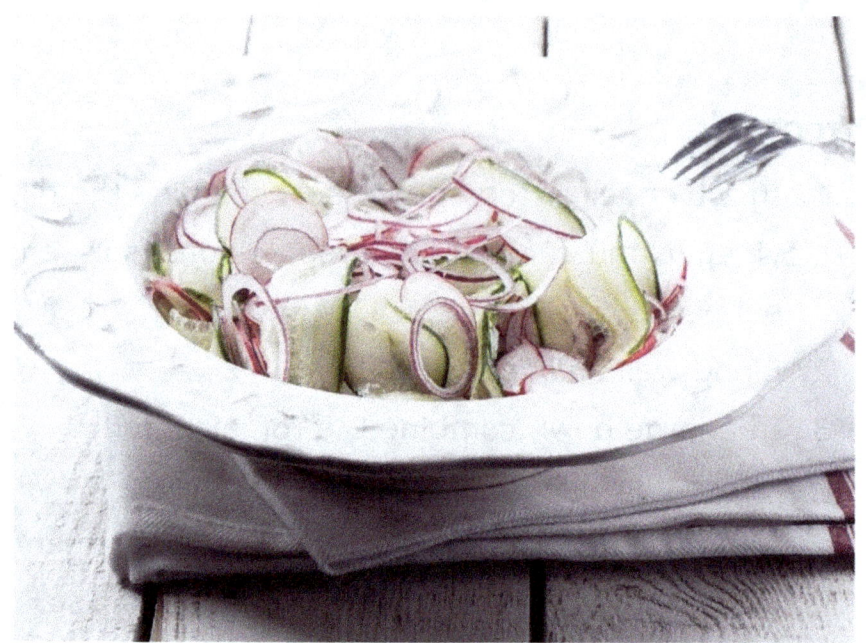

Preparation time: 15 minutes

cooking time: 0 minutes

servings: 4

Ingredients

- 2 medium English cucumbers, peeled, halved, seeded, cut into 1/4-inch slices

- 6 small red radishes, cut into 1/8-inch slices
- 1/2 teaspoon dried tarragon
- 2 1/2 tablespoons tarragon vinegar
- 1/4 teaspoon sugar
- Salt and freshly ground black pepper
- 1/4 cup olive oil

Directions

1. In a large bowl, combine the cucumbers and the radishes and set aside.
2. In a small bowl, combine the vinegar, tarragon, sugar, and salt and pepper to taste.
3. Whisk in the oil until well blended, then add the dressing to the salad.
4. Toss gently to combine and serve.

The Great Green Salad

Preparation Time: 10 Minutes

Cooking Time: 0 Minutes

Servings:

Ingredients

- 1 head Boston or Bibb lettuce
- 1 small zucchini, cut into ribbons with potato peeler
- 8 asparagus spears, trimmed and cut into 2-inch pieces
- 2 mini seedless cucumbers, sliced
- 1 avocado, peeled, pitted, and sliced
- ½ cup Green Goddess Dressing or store-bought vegan green goddess dressing
- 2 scallions, thinly sliced

Directions

1. Divide the lettuce leaves among 4 plates. Top each with some of the asparagus, cucumber, zucchini, and avocado.
2. Drizzle each bowl with 2 tablespoons of dressing and sprinkle with scallions.

Curried Fruit Salad

Preparation Time: 15 Minutes

Cooking Time: 0 Minutes

Servings: 4 To 6

Ingredients

- ¾ cup vegan vanilla yogurt
- 1/4 cup finely chopped mango chutney
- 1 tablespoon fresh lime juice
- 1 Fuji or Gala apple, cored and cut into 1/2-inch dice
- 2 ripe peaches, halved, pitted, and cut into 1/2-inch dice
- 4 ripe black plums, halved and cut into 1/4-inch slices
- 1 ripe mango, peeled, pitted, and cut into 1/2-inch dice
- 1 teaspoon mild curry powder
- 1 cup red seedless grapes, halved
- 1/4 cup unsweetened toasted shredded coconut
- 1/4 cup toasted slivered almonds

Directions

1. In a small bowl, combine the yogurt, chutney, lime juice, and curry powder and stir until well blended. Set aside.
2. In a large bowl, combine the apple, peaches, plums, mango, grapes, coconut, and almonds.
3. Add the dressing, toss gently to coat, and serve.

Potato Salad Redux

Preparation Time: 5 Minutes

Cooking Time: 30 Minutes

Servings: 4 To 6

Ingredients

- 1 1/2 pounds small white potatoes, unpeeled
- 2 celery ribs, cut into 1/4-inch slices
- 1/2 to ¾ cup vegan mayonnaise, homemade or store-bought
- 1/4 cup sweet pickle relish
- 3 tablespoons minced green onions
- 1 tablespoon soy milk
- 1 tablespoon tarragon vinegar
- 1 teaspoon Dijon mustard
- 1/2 teaspoon salt (optional)
- Freshly ground black pepper

Directions

1. In a large pot of salted boiling water, cook the potatoes until just tender, about 30 minutes.

2. Drain and set aside to cool. When cool enough to handle, peel the potatoes and cut them into 1-inch dice.
3. Transfer the potatoes to a large bowl and add the celery, pickle relish, and green onions. Set aside.
4. In a small bowl, combine the mayonnaise, soy milk, vinegar, mustard, salt, and pepper to taste.
5. Mix until well blended. Pour the dressing onto the potato mixture, toss gently to combine, and serve.

Brown Rice and Pepper Salad

Preparation Time: 15 Minutes

Cooking Time: 0 Minutes

Servings: 4

Ingredients

- 2 cups prepared brown rice
- ½ red onion, diced
- 1 red bell pepper, diced
- 2 tablespoons unseasoned rice vinegar
- 1 orange bell pepper, diced
- 1 carrot, diced
- ¼ cup olive oil
- 1 tablespoon soy sauce
- 1 garlic clove, minced
- 1 tablespoon grated fresh ginger
- ¼ teaspoon sea salt
- ¼ teaspoon freshly ground black pepper

Directions

1. In a large bowl, combine the rice, onion, bell peppers, and carrot.
2. In a small bowl, whisk together the olive oil, rice vinegar, soy sauce, garlic, ginger, salt, and pepper.
3. Toss with the rice mixture and serve immediately.

Radish and Walnuts Dip

Preparation time: 10 minutes

Cooking time: 20 minutes

Servings: 4

Ingredients:

- 2 tablespoons walnuts, chopped
- 4 scallions, chopped
- 2 tablespoons olive oil
- 1 cup coconut cream
- 2 cups radishes, chopped
- 1 teaspoon chili powder
- A pinch of salt and black pepper
- 2 teaspoons mustard powder
- 2 teaspoons garlic powder
- 2 teaspoons cumin, ground

Directions:

1. Heat up a pan with the oil over medium heat, add the scallions, mustard powder, garlic powder and cumin, stir and sauté for 5 minutes.

2. Add the walnuts, and the other ingredients, stir, cook over medium heat for 15 minutes.
3. Blend well using an immersion blender.
4. Divide into bowls and serve.

Nutrition:

Calories 192, fat 5, fiber 7, carbs 12, protein 5

Spinach and Artichoke Dip

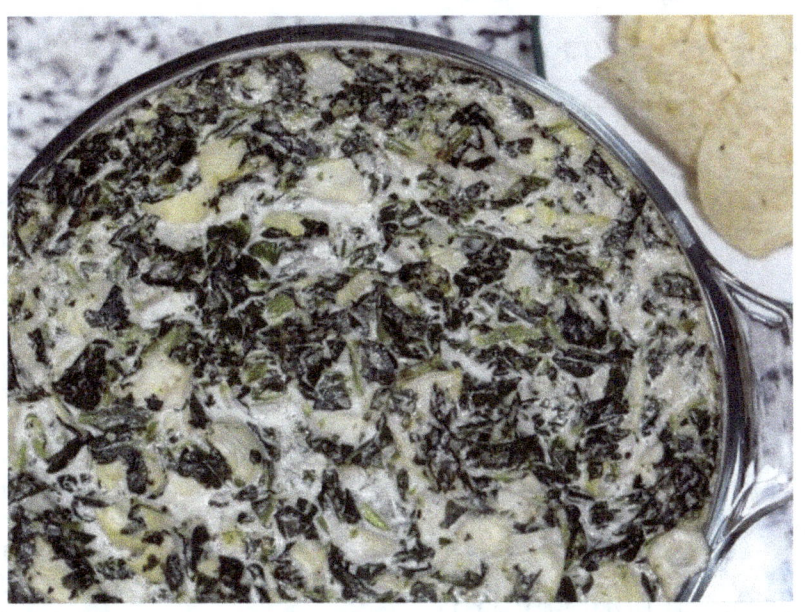

Preparation Time: 10 minutes

Cooking Time: 25 minutes

Servings: 10

Ingredients:

- 4 cups spinach
- 28 ounces artichokes
- 1 small white onion, peeled, diced
- 1 1/2 cups cashews, soaked, drained

- 1/4 cup nutritional yeast
- 4 cloves of garlic, peeled
- 1 1 1/2 teaspoons salt
- 1 tablespoon olive oil
- 2 tablespoons lemon juice
- 1 1/2 cups coconut milk, unsweetened

Directions:

1. Cook onion and garlic in hot oil for 3 minutes until saute and then set aside until required.
2. Place cashews in a food processor; add 1 teaspoon salt, yeast, milk, and lemon juice and pulse until smooth.
3. Add spinach, onion mixture, and artichokes and pulse until the chunky mixture comes together.
4. Tip the dip in a heatproof dish and bake for 20 minutes at 425 degrees f until the top is browned and dip bubbles.
5. Serve straight away with vegetable sticks.

Nutrition:

Calories:124 Cal, Fat: 9 g, Carbs: 8 g, Protein: 5 g, Fiber: 1 g

Chaffles With Raspberry Syrup

Preparation Time: 10 minutes

Cooking Time: 38 minutes

Servings: 4

Ingredients:

For the chaffles:

- 1 egg, beaten
- 1 tsp almond flour
- ½ cup finely shredded cheddar cheese
- 1 tsp sour cream

For the raspberry syrup:

- 1 cup fresh raspberries
- ¼ cup water
- ¼ cup swerve sugar
- 1 tsp vanilla extract

Directions:

For the chaffles:

1. Preheat the cast iron pan.
2. Meanwhile, in a medium bowl, mix the egg, cheddar cheese, almond flour, and sour cream.

3. Open the iron, pour in half of the mixture, cover, and cook until crispy, 7 minutes.
4. Remove the chaffle onto a plate and make another with the remaining batter.

For the raspberry syrup:

5. Meanwhile, add the raspberries, swerve sugar, water, and vanilla extract to a medium pot. Set over low heat and cook until the raspberries soften and sugar becomes syrupy. Occasionally stir while mashing the raspberries as you go. Turn the heat off when your desired consistency is achieved and set aside to cool.
6. Drizzle some syrup on the chaffles and enjoy when ready.

Nutrition:

Calories 105, Fats 7.11g, Carbs 4.31g, Net Carbs 2.21g, Protein 5.83g

Banana Chocolate Cupcakes

Preparation time: 20 minutes

cooking time: 20 minutes

servings: 12 cupcakes

Ingredients

- 3 medium bananas
- 2 tablespoons almond butter
- 1 cup non-dairy milk
- 1 teaspoon apple cider vinegar
- 1 teaspoon pure vanilla extract
- 1¼ cups whole-wheat flour
- ½ cup rolled oats
- ¼ cup coconut sugar (optional
- ½ teaspoon baking soda
- 1 teaspoon baking powder
- ½ cup unsweetened cocoa powder
- ¼ cup chia seeds, or sesame seeds
- Pinch sea salt
- ¼ cup dark chocolate chips, dried cranberries, or raisins (optional)

Directions

1. Preheat the oven to 350 °F. Lightly grease the cups of two 6-cup muffin tins or line with paper muffin cups.
2. Put the bananas, milk, almond butter, vinegar, and vanilla in a blender and purée until smooth. Or stir together in a large bowl until smooth and creamy.
3. Put the flour, oats, sugar (if using), baking powder, baking soda, cocoa powder, chia seeds, salt, and chocolate chips in another large bowl, and stir to combine. Mix together the wet and dry ingredients, stirring as little as possible. Spoon into muffin cups, and bake for 20 to 25 minutes. Take the cupcakes out of the oven and let them cool fully before taking out of the muffin tins, since they'll be very moist.

Nutrition (1 cupcake)

Calories: 215; Total fat: 6g; Carbs: 39g; Fiber: 9g; Protein: 6g

Mint Chocolate Chip Sorbet

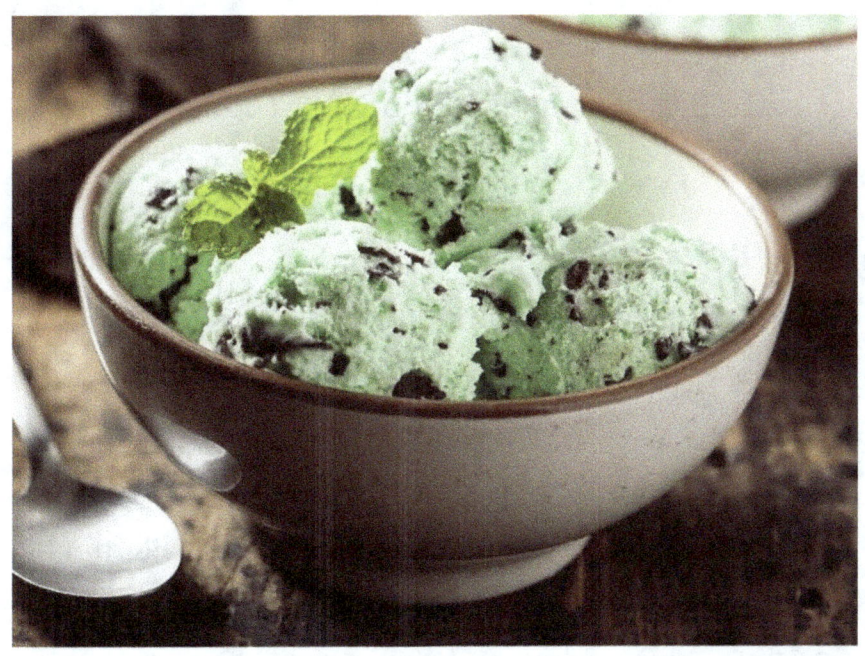

Preparation time: 5 minutes

cooking time: 0 minutes

servings: 1

Ingredients

- 1 frozen banana
- 1 tablespoon almond butter, or peanut butter, or other nut or seed butter

- 2 to 3 tablespoons non-dairy chocolate chips, or cocoa nibs
- 2 tablespoons fresh mint, minced
- ¼ cup or less non-dairy milk (only if needed)
- 2 to 3 tablespoons goji berries (optional)

Directions

1. Put the banana, almond butter, and mint in a food processor or blender and purée until smooth.
2. Add the non-dairy milk if needed to keep blending (but only if needed, as this will make the texture less solid).
3. Pulse the chocolate chips and goji berries (if using into the mix so they're roughly chopped up).

Nutrition

Calories: 212; Total fat: 10g; Carbs: 31g; Fiber: 4g; Protein: 3g

Pineapple and Melon Stew

Preparation time: 10 minutes

Cooking time: 15 minutes

Servings: 4

Ingredients:

- 2 tablespoons stevia
- 1 cup pineapple, peeled and cubed
- 1 cup melon, peeled and cubed
- 1 teaspoon vanilla extract
- 2 cups water

Directions:

1. In a pan, combine the pineapple with the melon and the other ingredients, toss gently, cook over medium-low heat for 15 minutes, divide into bowls and serve cold.

Nutrition:

Calories 40, fat 4.3, fiber 2.3, carbs 3.4, protein 0.8

Pumpkin Spice Oat Bars.

Preparation Time: 25 Minutes

Servings: 10

Ingredients:

- 2 cups old-fashioned rolled oats
- 2/3 cup canned solid-pack pumpkin
- 1 cup non-dairy milk
- ½ cup chopped toasted pecans
- ½ cup sweetened dried cranberries
- 6 ounces soft or silken tofu, drained and crumbled
- ½ cup packed light brown sugar or granulated natural sugar
- 2 teaspoons ground cinnamon
- 1½ teaspoons baking powder
- 1 teaspoon salt
- 1 teaspoon pure vanilla extract
- ¼ teaspoon ground nutmeg
- ¼ teaspoon ground allspice

Directions:

1. Lightly oil a baking tray that will fit in the steamer basket of your Cooker.
2. Stir together the oats, cinnamon, nutmeg, allspice, sugar, baking powder, and salt.
3. Blend together the tofu, pumpkin, milk, and vanilla until smooth and even.
4. Stir the wet and dry ingredients together before folding in the pecans and cranberries.
5. Pour the batter into your tray and put the tray in your steamer basket.
6. Pour the minimum amount of water into the base of your Cooker and lower the steamer basket.
7. Seal and cook on Steam for 12 minutes.
8. Release the pressure quickly and set to one side to cool a little before slicing.

Tutti Frutti Cobbler.

Preparation Time: 30 Minutes

Servings: 6

Ingredients:

- 1¼ cups unbleached all-purpose flour
- 1 cup fresh blueberries, rinsed and picked over
- 2 large ripe peaches, peeled, pitted, and sliced
- 1 cup fresh blackberries, rinsed and picked over
- ¾ cup natural sugar
- ½ cup unsweetened almond milk
- 2 ripe apricots, peeled, pitted, and sliced
- 1½ tablespoons tapioca starch or cornstarch
- 1 tablespoon vegetable oil
- 1 teaspoon baking powder
- ½ teaspoon pure vanilla extract
- ¼ teaspoon salt
- ¼ teaspoon ground cinnamon

Directions:

1. Lightly oil a baking tray that will fit in the steamer basket of your Cooker.

2. Toss the fruit in the tapioca and ½ a cup of sugar and put in the tray.
3. Put the tray in your steamer basket.
4. Pour the minimum amount of water into the base of your Cooker and lower the steamer basket.
5. Seal and cook on Steam for 12 minutes.
6. In a bowl stir together the flour, remaining sugar, cinnamon, baking powder, and salt.
7. Slowly combine with the almond milk, vanilla, and oil until soft dough is formed.
8. Release the Cooker's pressure quickly, give the fruit a stir, and cover with the dough.
9. Seal and Steam for another 5 minutes.
10. Release the pressure quickly and set to one side to cool a little.

Bread & Butter Pudding.

Preparation Time: 25 Minutes

Servings: 8

Ingredients:

- 3 cups nondairy milk, warmed
- 2 cups cubed spiced bread or cake, stale is better
- 1 (16-ouncecan solid-pack pumpkin
- 2 cups cubed whole-grain bread, stale is better
- 3 tablespoons rum or bourbon or 1 teaspoon rum extract (optional)
- ¾ cup packed light brown sugar or granulated natural sugar
- 1 teaspoon pure vanilla extract
- 1½ teaspoons ground cinnamon
- ¼ teaspoon ground nutmeg
- ¼ teaspoon ground allspice
- ¼ teaspoon ground ginger
- ¼ teaspoon salt

Directions:

1. Lightly oil a baking tray that will fit in the steamer basket of your Cooker.
2. Put the bread cubes in the tray.
3. Mix the pumpkin, sugar, vanilla, rum, spices, and salt.
4. Slowly stir in the milk.
5. Pour the mix over the bread.
6. Pour the minimum amount of water into the base of your Cooker and lower the steamer basket.
7. Seal and cook on Steam for 20 minutes.
8. Release the pressure quickly and set to one side to cool a little.

Pastry with Nuts, Mango and Blueberries

Preparation time: 45 minutes

Ingredients:

For the pastry:

- 1 cup whole wheat flour
- ½ cup whole wheat almond flour
- 12 Oz. blueberries or any berries to your liking
- 2 Mangoes
- ½ cup butter
- 2 eggs yolks
- 2 Oz. water
- 1 pinch of pumpkin seeds
- Sesame and sunflower seeds
- Peanuts, dried

For the filling:

- 8 Oz. cream cheese
- 1 mango, chopped
- 2 tbsp. lemon juice
- ½ icing sugar

Directions:

1. In a bowl mix the flour ingredients with the butter, add the egg yolks and some water until combined and forms a ball.
2. Knead the dough a little until it is smooth and refrigerate for half an hour covered with a napkin.
3. Mix all the ingredients of the pastry filling in a blender.
4. Grease your baking tray or a cooking tin and dust with some flour.
5. Pour the dough into the tin and bake for 30 minutes (200 grades) until lightly brown.
6. Pour the filling onto the pastry and top it with berries and nuts. Add some dessert sauce for serving.

Cashew Fudge

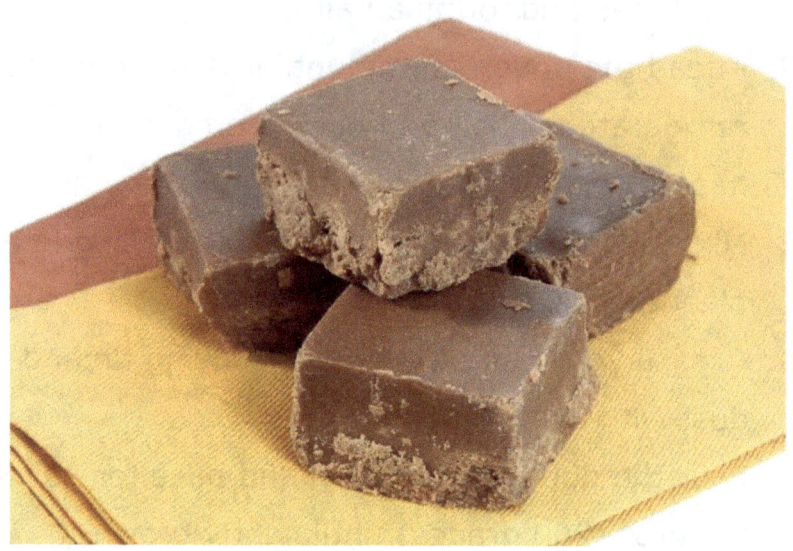

Preparation time: 3 hours

Cooking time: 0 minutes

Servings: 6

Ingredients:

- 1/3 cup cashew butter
- ½ cup cashews, soaked for 8 hours and drained
- 1 cup coconut cream
- 5 tablespoons lime juice

- ½ teaspoon lime zest, grated
- 1 tablespoons stevia

Directions:

1. In a bowl, mix the cashew butter with the cream, the cashews and the other ingredients and whisk well.
2. Line a muffin tray with parchment paper, scoop 1 tablespoon of the fudge mix in each of the muffin tins and freeze for 3 hours before serving.

Nutrition:

Calories 200, fat 4.5, fiber 3.4, carbs 13.5, protein 5

Raisins and Berries Cream

Preparation time: 5 minutes

Cooking time: 0

Servings: 4

Ingredients:

- 1 cup coconut cream
- 1 cup blackberries
- 2 tablespoons raisins
- 3 tablespoons stevia
- 2 tablespoons lime juice

Directions:

1. In a blender, the cream with the berries and the other ingredients except the raisins, pulse well, divide into cups, sprinkle the raisins on top and cool down before serving.

Nutrition:

Calories 192, fat 6.5, fiber 3.4, carbs 9.5, protein 5

Avocado and Grapes Shake Bowls

Preparation time: 5 minutes

Cooking time: 0 minutes

Servings: 4

Ingredients:

- 2 avocados, peeled, pitted and chopped
- 1 cup grapes, halved
- ¾ cup almond milk
- ½ teaspoon vanilla extract
- Juice of 1 lime

Directions:

1. In a blender, combine the avocados with the grapes and the other ingredients, pulse well, divide into bowls and serve cold.

Nutrition:

Calories 328, fat 30.4, fiber 8, carbs 16.1, protein 3.1

Avocado Cookies

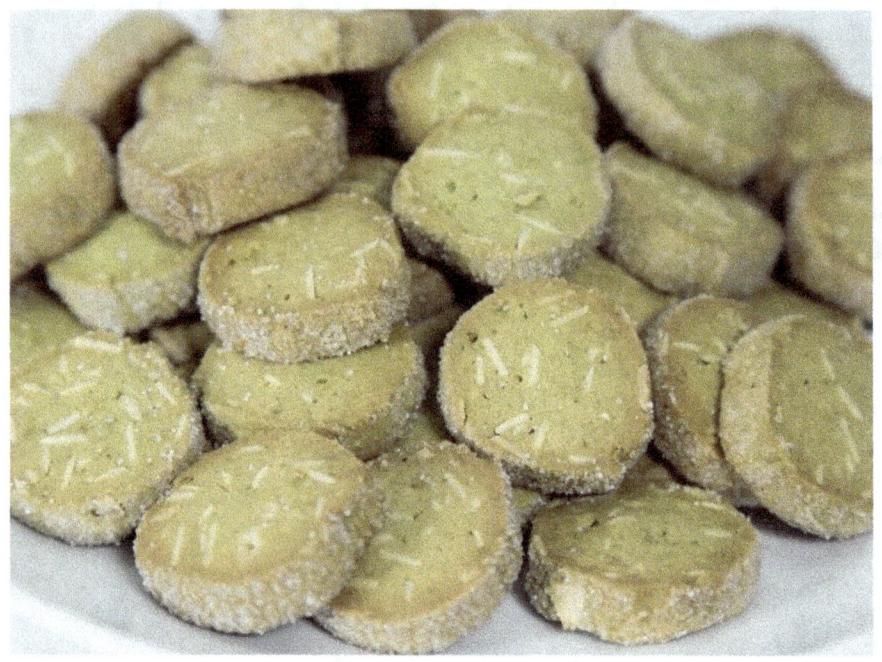

Preparation time: 10 minutes

Cooking time: 20 minutes

Servings: 10

Ingredients:

- 1 cup avocado, peeled, pitted and mashed
- 2 tablespoons flaxseed mixed with 3 tablespoons water

- 2 cups coconut flour
- 1 teaspoon vanilla extract
- 1 teaspoon baking powder
- 1 cup avocado oil
- ½ cup stevia
- 1 cup coconut, unsweetened and shredded

Directions:

1. In a bowl, combine the flour with the avocado, the flaxseed and the other ingredients, and whisk really well.
2. Scoop tablespoons of dough on a baking sheet lined with parchment paper, flatten them, introduce them in the oven at 350 degrees F and bake for 20 minutes.
3. Leave the cookies to cool down and serve.

Nutrition:

Calories 200, fat 4.5, fiber 3.4, carbs 9.5, protein 2.4

Rice Pudding

Preparation time: 10 minutes

Cooking time: 20 minutes

Servings: 4

Ingredients:

- ½ cup avocado, peeled, pitted and cubed
- 1 cup cauliflower rice
- 2 cups coconut milk
- 1 cup coconut cream
- 1 teaspoon vanilla extract
- 1 tablespoon cinnamon powder
- ½ cup stevia

Directions:

1. In a pot, mix the cauliflower rice with the milk, the cream and the other ingredients, stir, bring to a simmer and cook for 20 minutes.
2. Divide into bowls and serve.

Nutrition:

Calories 234, fat 9.5, fiber 3.4, carbs 12.4, protein 6.5

Strawberry Sorbet

Preparation time: 3 hours

Cooking time: 10 minutes

Servings: 4

Ingredients:

- 2 cups coconut water
- 1 teaspoon vanilla extract
- 1 teaspoon lime zest, grated
- 1 pound strawberries, halved
- 1 cup stevia

Directions:

1. Heat up a pan with the coconut water over medium heat, add berries, stevia and the other ingredients, whisk, simmer for 10 minutes, transfer to a blender, pulse, divide into bowls and keep in the freezer for 3 hours before serving.

Nutrition:

Calories 182, fat 5.4, fiber 3.4, carbs 12, protein 5.4

Coconut Cream

Preparation time: 5 minutes

Cooking time: 0 minutes

Servings: 2

Ingredients:

- 2 cups coconut cream
- 2 cups coconut flesh, unsweetened shredded
- 3 tablespoons mint, chopped
- 2 tablespoons stevia
- ½ teaspoon cocoa powder

Directions:

1. In a blender, combine the coconut flesh with the mint, the cream and the other ingredients, pulse well, divide into cups and serve cold.

Nutrition:

Calories 193, fat 5.4, fiber 3.4, carbs 7.6, protein 3

Brown Fat Bombs

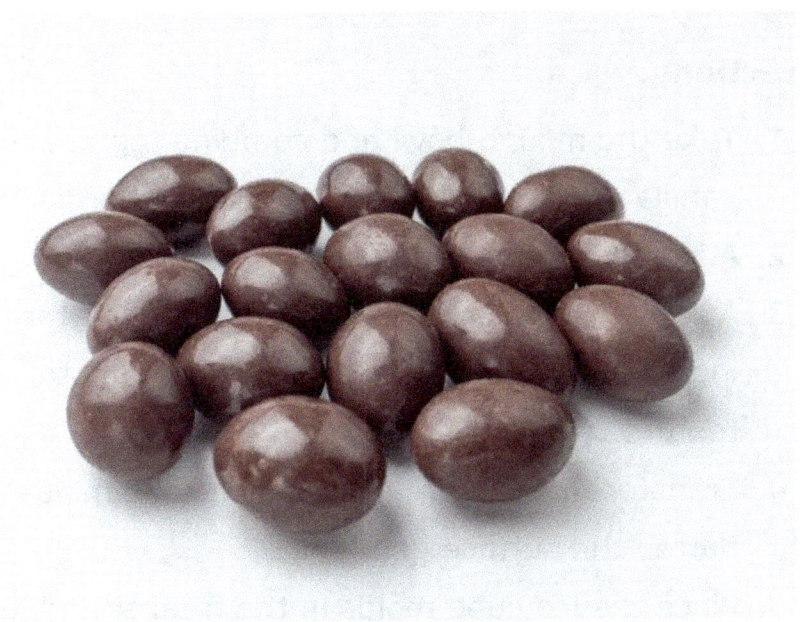

Preparation time: 7 minutes

Cooking time: 30 minutes

Servings: 2

Ingredients:

- 2 tablespoon cocoa powder
- 1 teaspoon vanilla extract
- 1/3 teaspoon instant coffee
- 1 tablespoon liquid stevia

- ¾ teaspoon salt
- 1/3 cup coconut butter

Directions:

1. Take the mixing bowl and combine together vanilla extract, liquid stevia, and instant coffee.
2. Add salt and melted butter.
3. After this, add cocoa powder and mix up the ingredients until you get a soft and smooth texture.
4. Transfer the mixture into the ice cube molds and flatten the surface gently.
5. Place the ice cube molds in the freezer and let them stay there for 30 minutes.

Nutrition:

Calories 266, fat 24.7, fiber 8.3, carbs 12.6, protein 3.7

Nut Fudge

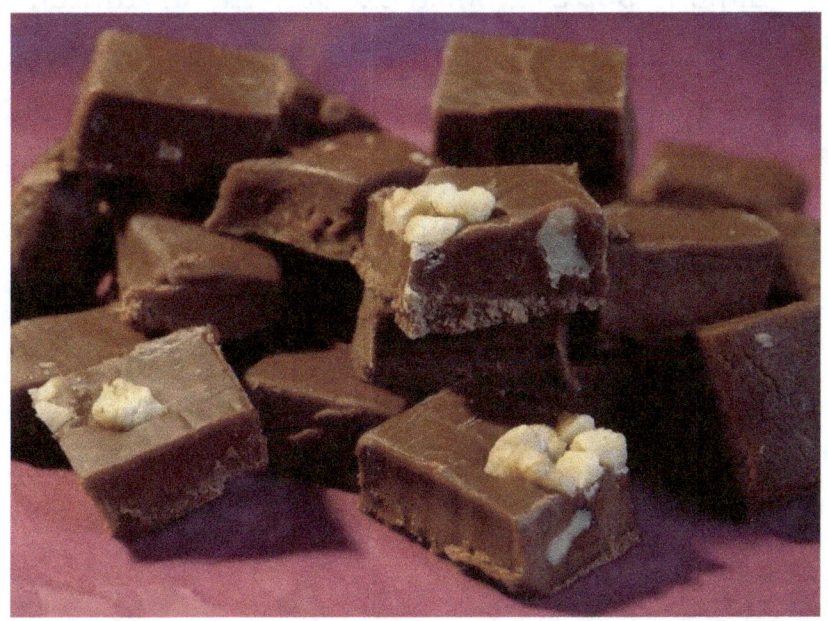

Preparation time: 8 minutes

Cooking time: 1.5 hours

Servings: 3

Ingredients:

- 1 tablespoon almonds, crushed
- ½ teaspoon vanilla extract
- 4 tablespoon almond butter
- 1 tablespoon Erythritol

Directions:

1. Take the mixing bowl and combine in it the almond butter, vanilla extract, and Erythritol.
2. Transfer the bowl on the water bath, start to preheat it, and stir gently.
3. When the mixture is homogenous – add crushed almonds, stir it, and remove from the water bath.
4. Place the butter mixture in the mini muffin molds and transfer in the freezer.
5. Freeze it for 1.5 hours.

Nutrition:

Calories 144, fat 13, fiber 2.4, carbs 9.5, protein 5

Quick Choco Brownie

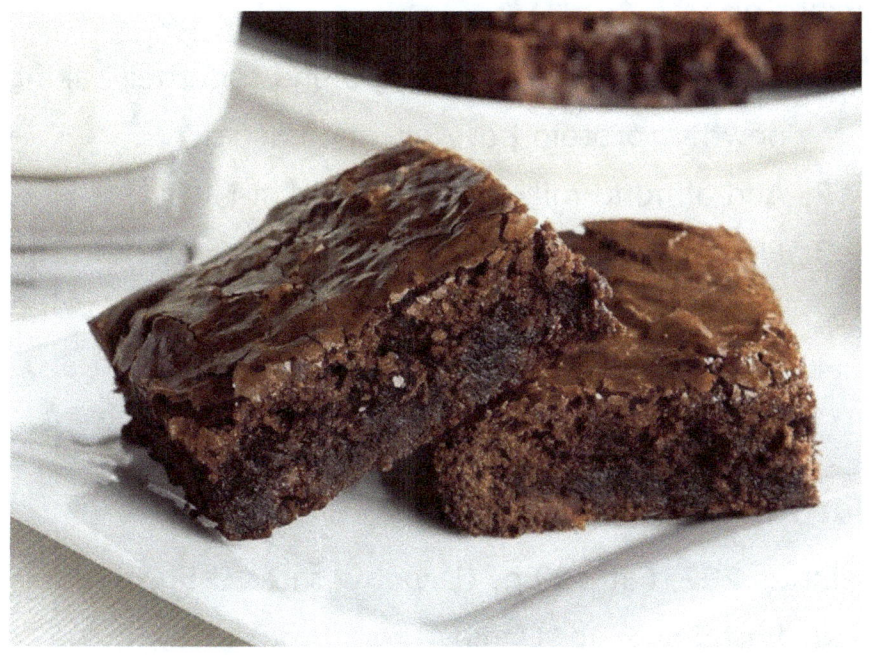

Preparation Time: 10 minutes

Cooking Time: 0 minute

Servings: 1

Ingredients:

- 1 tbsp cocoa powder
- 1/4 cup almond milk
- 1 scoop chocolate protein powder

- 1/2 tsp baking powder

Directions:

1. In a microwave-safe mug blend together baking powder, protein powder, and cocoa.
2. Add almond milk in a mug and stir well.
3. Place mug in microwave and microwave for 30 seconds.
4. Serve and enjoy.

Nutrition:

Calories 207, Fat 15.8g, Carbohydrates 9.5g, Sugar 3.1g, Protein 12.4g, Cholesterol 20mg

NOTE

www.ingramcontent.com/pod-product-compliance
Lightning Source LLC
Chambersburg PA
CBHW070931080526
44589CB00013B/1480